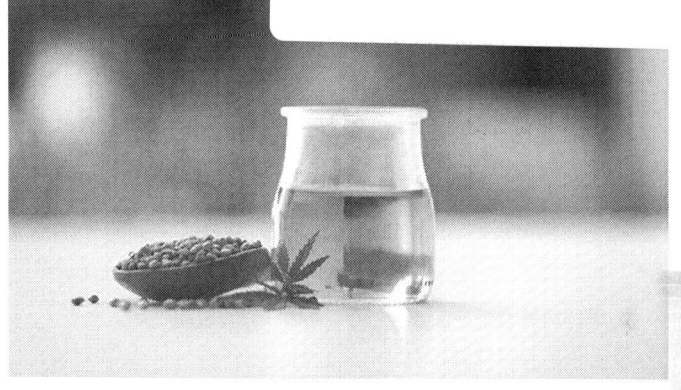

Hemp oil and CBD oil are rising in the ranks of the holistic, medicinal, and nutritional worlds, and for good reason. They're sourced in plants, ensuring that they're completely natural, without any of the chemicals in current health products, such as creams, body butters, and pain-management medicines (all things these oils can replace). Essentially, a look at the hemp plant is a look at a medicinal bounty, one that we've been avoiding for too long, given its association with drug culture.

Of course, beating back against preconceived notions of the culture behind the hemp plant can be difficult. This is because hemp, the plant from which both are taken, is indeed the very source of marijuana and "illicit" drug use. But in fact, CBD and hemp oil have no association to the negative sides of drug use. Rather, they can open up your body to incredible, natural, and plant-based benefits. They can give you new life.

In this book, we'll dive into the complex and dynamic world of getting nutritional and health benefits from hemp oil and CBD oil. As you're about to discover, hemp oil and CBD oil are only cousins—derived from very different parts of the plant. And because of their differences, they deliver very different benefits to your body.

Essentially, hemp oil is better utilized for nutritional and beauty-based resources, while CBD is more impactful, allowing for pain management, assisting with everything from arthritis pain to migraines to anxiety and even depression and schizophrenia. This book utilizes science-backed examples to prove that CBD oil is a dramatic and impactful way to rejuvenate your health. In fact, many studies have shown that it can be as beneficial as certain kinds of medicines. In a world where we pop pills, day after day, not thinking about the consequences, it could be beneficial to consider how best to restructure our pain management plans for a more environmental approach.

Doctors and scientists everywhere seem to agree.

Once it names the benefits of hemp oil and CBD oil, the book goes on to tell you how you can actually make your own—squeezing the oil from the seeds, and taking it from the actual plant. It also gives you recommendations for purchasing, if you don't want to make it at home (which is reasonable, as it can become expensive and time-consuming). It further gives you information about dosing your CBD oil, as it should be handled with care, despite its lack of toxicity.

Furthermore, you'll find beauty and food-related hemp oil recipes, allowing you to reap the rewards of the gorgeous and nutritional oil, without simply eating it plain (it kind of tastes like olive oil, FYI).

This is the everything you need to know, no questions asked, health book about hemp oil and CBD oil. And, if you follow along closely, it will set you free—allowing you to take charge of your health and rejuvenate your mind. Soon, you won't be latched into a world of medication and too many doctor's bills. Who knew, that a simple plant might give us all the fuel we need to survive.

TABLE OF CONTENTS

CHAPTER 1: 9
CHAPTER 2: 15
CHAPTER 3: 27
Chapter 4: 37
Chapter 5: 53

Chapter 6: 61
HEMP OIL AND GARLIC DRESSING 63
PESTO WITH HEMPSEED 64
CREAMY SALAD DRESSING WITH HEMP 65
HEMP SEED VINAIGRETTE FOR SALADS 66
HEMP OIL HUMMUS 67
HEMP AND CHOCOLATE SMOOTHIE 68
PURPLE BERRY HEMP OIL SMOOTHIE 69
GREEN HEMP OIL SMOOTHIE 70

HEMP OIL FOR BEAUTY AND SKIN CARE 71
ANTI-ECZEMA HEALING BODY BUTTER 77
FOREST FOR THE TREES BALM 78
HEALING LIP BALM 79
HEMP OIL FACE MASK WITH AVOCADO 80
HEMP OIL SOAP 81

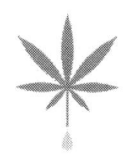

CHAPTER 1:
Hemp Oil and CBD Explained

What's the difference between CBD oil and hemp oil? Often, they're used interchangeably and incorrectly (usually, just by people who want to talk about their drug-based association, who want to run away from anything called "hemp").

Yes, they're taken from the same marijuana plant, and the same plant as one another. But the difference lies in where these compounds are derived from. The seeds of the plant, or the plant itself?

Read on for a breakdown of where these oils come from, and how they're generally used to benefit daily life.

WHAT IS HEMP OIL?

Hemp oil is an extract from the seeds of the hemp plant. This type of oil can actually be taken from all the seeds of plants in the cannabis realm, but we only really get hemp oil from industrial plants. This means that the amount of "psychoactive" substances is reduced and regulated—and it won't affect you like any "high" might.

HOW CAN YOU USE HEMP OIL?

Hemp oil is an incredible ingredient for foods and recipes, including salads and pastas. It offers a bit of a nutty flair, along with a crispness, which is often chosen over olive oil when cooking. And as the benefits are further-reaching than olive oil, in many capacities, it's a good substitution to make. More on that later.

Instead of petroleum, hemp oil can actually be used to make certain types of plastics. This would make our plastic use more environmentally friendly, and help us move away from using fossil fuels. Using petroleum—a source that we literally cannot make more of—is always irresponsible. And we must find better ways to produce and reuse and grow.

In fact, Hemp Plastic is affordable, and completely natural, meaning that it will be broken down in nature after use—much like vegetables in the compost. Hemp plastic can be used to make paints, smartphones, toys, railways, household items such as plants, socks, and cookware—which means growing hemp is actually a responsible way to move forward in our exploration of more environmentally friendly ways to live and work and use resources.

Also, hemp oil is an incredible natural moisturizer, which many women use in the shower for cleansing, reducing wrinkles, and fighting acne. In fact, it has a compound that ensures it doesn't clog your pores, making it an essential part of every woman's everyday moisturizing and cleansing regime. And because it's cheaper than buying separate ointments and creams for separate facial cleanings, moisturizing sessions, and even strengthening your cuticles, there's no reason you shouldn't learn to incorporate it into your routine. We'll have some recipes at the end of this book.

Hemp oil can also be used as a bio-diesel fuel, meaning that it can literally take us places, while keeping the world environmentally safe and conscious. All that power in a single plant. Why aren't people paying more attention?

WHAT IS CBD OIL?

Rather than being extracted from the seed of the hemp plant, CBD oil is made from the stalks, the leaves, and the flowers of the hemp plant. CBD is short for "cannabidiol, which at one time was just known as a tiny molecule in the hemp plant—before becoming a recent transformational part of the nutrition and medical industry, after years of research.

Cannabidiol is an incredibly important part of the medical marijuana industry, as it takes on all the benefits of medical marijuana, without all the side effects of smoking a typical blunt. In fact, despite being the second most common cannabinoid in the hemp plant, it is non-psychotropic and will not offer a high.

The uses of CBD oil are even more impressive than hemp oil. In fact, CBD oil can be used to treat cancer. It's also used for the treatment of anxiety, inflammation, seizures, depression, and other neuro disorders. Beyond that, it's also been used for the treatment of epilepsy, which causes seizures.

WHAT'S THE DIFFERENCE BETWEEN HEMP OIL AND CBD OIL, THEN?

Essentially, the properties of CBD oil and hemp oil make them incredibly different for everyday use. Hemp oil is filled with nutrients, and can be used for eco-friendly plant production and creating lotions and soaps. It's perfect for cooking, and is a beneficial part of every diet. CBD oil, on the other hand, has significantly higher amount of cannabidiol in it, due to being taken from the flowers, stalks, and leaves of hemp plants. It's used in the treatment of cancers, for anxiety and depression, and for other ailments—meaning it's more medicinal in nature than hemp oil.

So therefore, if someone tells you that hemp oil is beneficial for medicinal reasons, they're lying—but they have good intentions in mind. But if someone tries to tell you that hemp oil and CBD oil are filled with THC—the stuff that makes you high—they're absolutely incorrect. Marijuana has a much higher THC count than hemp. And it's a means to a good party, maybe, rather than a more thoughtful and progressive and healthful life.

Read on to the next chapter for the health benefits of hemp oil, and how it can lead you toward a more nutritional life, both in the kitchen and out.

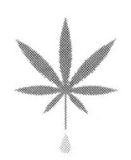

CHAPTER 2:
Hemp Oil Benefits

Hemp oil is a well-documented nutritional oil, which can be used for beauty and dietary needs. Unlike its brother, "hash oil," which is used to make things like pot brownies and high cookies, it doesn't get you "high" in the traditional, marijuana sense, which makes it a beneficial part of everyday life.

You must know, however, that any claims that hemp oil can be used to cure cancer aren't backed up by science. We'll have more on that later, while discussing CBD—its more powerful cousin.

WHY IS HEMP OIL HEALTHY?

Hemp seeds contain an incredible amount of nutrients, including omega 6 fatty acids, polynunsaturated fatty acids, protein, vitamin E antioxidants (which, yes, can lead to a decreased risk of cancer), omega 3 fatty acids, insoluble fiber, along with iron, potassium, magnesium, zinc, phosphorus, calcium, linoleic acid, and even various microelements, like chromium.

THE TOP HEALTH BENEFITS OF HEMP OIL INCLUDE:

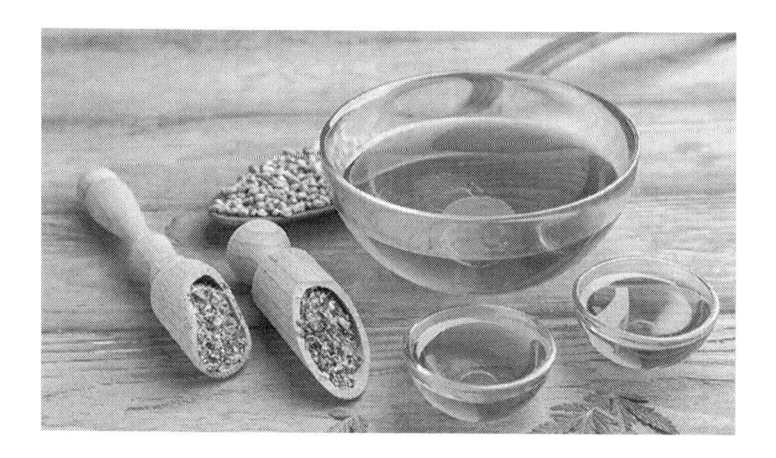

Growth of New Skin Cells, Fighting Aging

The linoleic acid in hemp oil has been proven to promote the growth of new skin cells, while fighting skin irritation, such as that caused by psoriasis and eczema.

Essential for Vegetarians and Vegans

Hemp oil is essential for vegetarians and vegans as it promotes an increased intake of omega-6 fatty acids and omega-3 fatty acids, which are not typically found in a traditional vegetarian and vegan diet.

Know that your body cannot produce these fatty acids naturally, and therefore must get them from your foods.

Reduce Chronic Nerve Pain

Omega 6 fatty acids have incredible benefits, including helping to reduce chronic nerve pain.

Decrease Inflammation

Omega 6 fatty acids further help fight bodily inflammation. That's important, as inflammation can lead to things like heart disease, arthritis, diabetes, and Alzheimer's disease. Omega 6 fatty acids can further help treat arthritis, with some studies proving that morning stiffness and morning pain in the joints can decrease with an increase in this single nutrient.

Furthermore, omega 6 fatty acid have been proven to fight the aging process, beating back against wrinkles and promoting the formation of new skin cells.

Decrease Symptoms of ADHD

Hemp oil has also been shown to decrease the symptoms of ADHD, or attention deficit disorder, which affects everyone from children to adults, interrupting their lives and disallowing mindful organization. According to a study that studied children between the ages of 8 and 18 years old, more than a quarter of the subjects experienced a reduction in ADHD symptoms after just a few months of using hemp oil. And after six months, nearly half of those in the experiment experienced a decrease in ADHD symptoms.

Omega 3 fatty acids, also found in hemp oil, match omega 6 fatty acids in their importance.

Fight Depression and Anxiety

For one, studies show that people who take more omega 3 fatty acids are less depressed and anxious. Some studies have even shown that omega 3 fatty acids are just as powerful as the anti-depression pill, Prozac. This could mean that hemp oil could replace some of your medications—freeing you from unnecessary medical bills.

Fight Blindness

Omega 3 fatty acids can further boost your eye health, and fight potential blindness.

Boost Baby's Brain Development If Pregnant

Furthermore, if you're pregnant, the omega 3 fatty acids in hemp oil can boost your baby's brain development. According to scientists, omega 3 fatty acids are associated with better communicative skills in children, a decreased risk of developing things like autism and ADHD, and even an increased intelligence.

Boost Heart Health

Despite the fact that "fat" is associated with poor heart health, omega 3 fatty acids are actually known to benefit heart health, causing a reduction in triglycerides, lowering of your blood pressure, decreasing the plaque on your arteries, decreasing your blood platelets from clumping together, and, again, decreasing inflammation.

Decrease Symptoms of Metabolic Syndrome

Also, omega 3 fatty acids have been shown to reduce symptoms of metabolic syndrome. Metabolic syndrome includes such conditions as high blood pressure, a resistance to insulin (which can lead to rapid weight gain and diabetes), belly fat (which is the most dangerous kind), and heart disease. Essentially, metabolic syndrome first makes you uncomfortably overweight, and then doesn't allow your body to fight it off through exercise. It can be a death sentence, if you don't work to fight it with nutrition.

Decrease Mental Disorders and Mood Swings

Omega 3 fatty acids have also been shown to decrease mental disorders, such as mood swings that are related to bipolar disorder and schizophrenia. Furthermore, if you increase your omega 3 fatty acids, you could reduce your risk for violent episodes, if these are a problem in your life.

Prevent Certain Kinds of Cancers

While hemp oil isn't a treatment for cancer, the omega 3 fatty acids have been proven to prevent certain types of cancers, with studies showing that people who eat more omega 3 fatty acids have up to 55% decreased risk of colon cancer. Omega 3 fatty acids have further been linked to a decreased risk of breast cancer and prostate cancer.

Decrease Your Menstrual Symptoms

For women, hemp oil's omega 3 fatty acids have further been shown to decrease your menstrual pain, the cramps and aches that occur in your lower back and in your pelvis. According to several studies, women who consume more omega 3 fatty acids actually have a decreased response to their period pain. A few studies have even shown that omega 3 fatty acids are more beneficial for period pain than ibuprofen.

Increase Your Ability To Sleep

Also, omega 3 fatty acids have been shown to boost your ability to sleep through the night. A lack of sleep is one of the most common reasons for several bodily imbalances, that which can lead to diabetes, depression, and even obesity. When you take in more omega 3 fatty acids, you increase your level of melatonin, which helps you fall asleep and fall into deeper sleep—that which helps your body repair itself, and reduces brain inflammation which can lead to future disorders, like depression.

Manage the Oils In Your Skin

Furthermore, omega 3 fatty acids may be responsible for the healthy structure of your skin cells. When you have healthy skin cells, they're moist and soft and wet, not the dry cells that lead to wrinkles. With more omega 3 fatty acids, you can boost the hydration in your skin, boost the production of oils, prevent the "red dots" that occur on your skin that are cosmetically ugly, not to mention painful, and even prevent acne.

Also, amazingly, the omega 3 fatty acids have a hand in fighting back against skin damage, as it blocks the release of the particles that actually eat your skin's collagen after you get a bit too much sun.

Balance Blood Sugar

Furthermore, hemp oil can help to balance out blood sugar, which makes it a beneficial part of any diabetic's diet. It's very low in carbohydrates, which ensures that it doesn't spike your insulin levels when you ingest it.

Reduce The Appearance of Varicose Veins

Varicose veins can ruin your look, disallowing you from things like skirts and dresses and shorts. But with the high omega 3 concentration in hemp oil, you can help thin out your blood, ensuring that it doesn't clot and form into varicose veins.

Hemp Oil Can Balance Your Hormones

Out of all the edible seeds in the universe (pine nuts, almonds, etc.), hemp seeds are the only ones that contain gamma-linolenic acid. This acid is eventually converted to the hormone called prostaglandin PGE1. This supports hormonal balance.

Imbalanced hormones is one of the most common health-related problems that women experience, especially during puberty, menopause, and perimenopause. It can be caused for many reasons, including taking in toxins (which are all around us, environmentally and in our foods), or just by living a lifestyle without balance. With unbalanced hormones, women can have an increased risk of certain types of breast cancers, and a boost in belly fat among other conditions.

Precautions When Using Hemp Oil

Of course, as with anything, hemp oil should be taken with precaution.

As mentioned previously, hemp oil has an ability to reduce clotting in your blood, which is good for some— but not for those who are taking blood thinners already. You might be one of these people if you have heart disease. Make sure you check your prescriptions!

Also, hemp oil allows for a boost in cell creation— which is beneficial for many cosmetic and health reasons. However, as hemp oil allows for rapid cell re-creation, it could promote the creation of prostate cancer. Therefore, if you have a history of prostate cancer in your family, it's important that you stay away from hemp oil or that you consult with your doctor prior to using it.

When consuming hemp oil, you shouldn't heat it. This will denature the unsaturated fats of the hemp oil, which makes it less healthy than in its current form.

Furthermore, if you take in too much hemp oil, it can lead to stomach cramps, diarrhea, or nausea. It shouldn't be taken in high amounts, and should be used with thought and diligence. This means that you should keep hemp oil away from children.

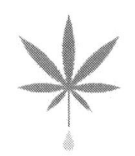

CHAPTER 3:
CBD Health Benefits

As mentioned, CBD is one of over sixty of the elements found in cannabis, which are then classified as cannabinoids. For the past several decades, THC—or tetrahydrocannabinol—was the main player in cannabis, as it's the one that produces the mind-bending "highs" for which cannabis is known. However, CBD is becoming a main player in the medicinal world, offering far more benefits than its THC brother.

CBD has no psychoactive compounds whatsoever. And according to many different studies over the years, its benefits include antioxidants, ant-inflammation, anxiolytic, amongst others—and can lead to benefiting everything from vomiting and anxiety to things like bipolar disorder and cancer.

Beyond that, CBD is just a different sort of cannabinoid in the hemp plant. The cannabinoids, on a molecular level, are known as "ligands," which essentially means they latch onto body proteins and then can alter the receptor from there, altering the behavior of cells. Unlike other cannabinoids, the receptors that allow CBD to latch onto them are mostly in the brain. Most of these receptors have to do with things like emotion, perception of the external world, cognition, hormonal functionality, and others. This means CBD has more power, on an emotional and brain level, than most cannabinoids.

Interestingly, the marijuana that's grown for recreational purposes is incredibly high in THC, and is lower in CBD. This means that smoking weed for recreational purposes doesn't necessarily lead to any of the following CBD-related benefits.

HEALTH BENEFITS OF CBD

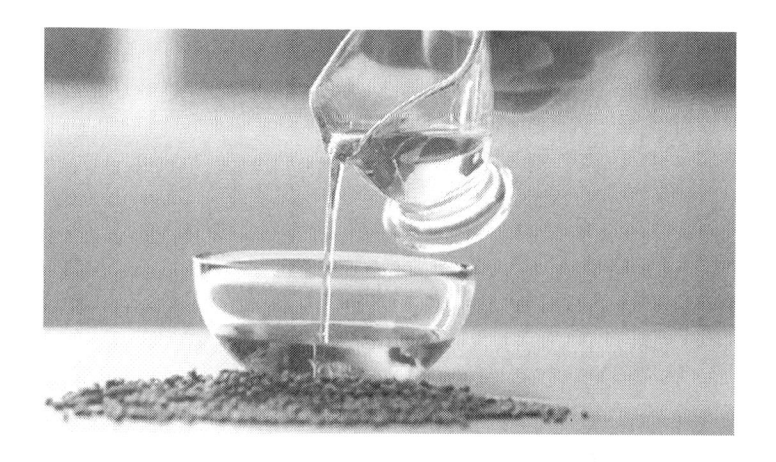

Can Be Used As An Antipsychotic

Whereas many people must seek out serious medication and drugs for psychotic problems, CBD has been shown to have antipsychotic effects. This is because it has a similar pharmacological profile to those drugs that are normally prescribed in such situations. Furthermore, when CBD has been used in actual cases, studies have shown that it prevents human psychosis and often helps relieve the side effects of schizophrenia. It's been shown to do this safely, without additional side effects.

Can Be Used To Help Fight Cancer

Back in 2006, a study from the Journal of Pharmacology and Experimental Therapeutics found that CBD could actually select specific breast cancer tumor cells and then stop the growth of them. This was huge, showing that it was potent against the generation of these new cells. Beyond that, further scientific studies showed that CBD could help to stop cancer cells from moving around the body, and from invading healthy cells.

CBD has also been shown that it could be effective to stop lung and colon cancer cells. It further contains properties that make it anti-tumor growth in gliomas. It's also been utilized in the treatment of leukemia, making it a powerful medicine in the game of cancer.

Furthermore, CBD is a non-toxin, with many studies showing that people who took in 700 mg of the oil every single day for six weeks didn't have any toxicity.

Can Help to Reduce Anxiety

CBD has been proven to alter the way the brain handles serotonin, which is a chemical that makes you feel happy. In fact, a study recently found that when people were given 600 mg of CBD right before giving a speech, the people were found to have less anxiety and performed much better.

Other studies, which were all conducted with animals, showed that CBD can be helpful in reducing stress that's associated with anxiety and ensuring that your heart rate doesn't get too high, which can be a cyclical problem that leads to increased anxiety. CBD was also shown to decrease the symptoms of post-traumatic stress disorder, or PTSD. Furthermore, CBD was shown to increase the ability to sleep, decreasing risk of insomnia.

Also, CBD was shown to be a helpful aid with things like obsessive compulsive disorder and panic disorder, amongst others.

In essence, if you struggle with anxiety, CBD can play an essential role in helping you get your life back.

Can Decrease Inflammation and Pain

As we get older, aches, pains and inflammation crop up from time to time, debilitate us, and make our lives just a little less colorful. However, one of CBD's best benefits is that it's a natural pain reliever. According to science, CBD is best used for handling pain because it actually inhibits certain brain pathways that are telling you you're in "serious pain."

Furthermore, a study from the Journal of Experimental Medicine found that CBD was also the root cause of suppressing certain brain pathways, while also suppressing inflammation. This means it helps to heal you, while making you stop feeling that which is ailing you.

Another study conducted back in 2007 showed that when CBD was combined with THC, it was often effective in the treatment of multiple sclerosis. As most multiple sclerosis patients suffer daily with serious pain, this could be revolutionary.

CBD Could Treat Neurological Disorders Like Seizures

Seizures are a huge issue for many children and adults, keeping them from normal activities, like driving cars or operating machinery. Seizures seemingly come out of nowhere, similar to a weather pattern. When they strike, anything could happen to the ailing person. This makes it incredibly important to figure out a way to beat them.

In a 2014 study, Stanford investigated children who experienced seizures. Nineteen were currently using CBD cannabis to treat them. Of that amount, 84% of the children experienced a decrease in frequency of seizures after using the cannabis with CBD. Of those people who experienced a decrease, 11% actually had a complete remission.

Furthermore, these children reported that they could sleep better, had better alertness, and were in a better mood as a result of the CBD. The side effects that they reported included being just kind of sleepy—which isn't a bad trade off.

Also that same year, there was another study that involved children who had epilepsy that was said to be resistant to treatment. The children received a CBD extract that was 98% oil-based. This was called Epidiolex.

After several months of this oil treatment, the patients reported back their results. Amazingly, 40% of the patients experienced a deceased amount of seizures by more than 50%.

In addition, animal studies that link epilepsy and CBD are very positive. CBD is generally non-toxic, and can be tolerated in children at a rate of about 25 milligrams per kilogram of a person's weight.

Can Boost Heart Health

According to a study from the British Journal of Clinical Pharmacology, CBD can protect against the kind of vascular damage that's normally created after eating too much sugar and is often seen in people with diabetes. Furthermore, CBD was shown to decrease something called vascular hyper permeability. This is something that causes leaky gut syndrome.

Shown To Reduce Nausea Symptoms

For hundreds of years, the cannabis plant has been utilized to decrease nausea and vomiting. But only recently have we really discovered just why this works.

Studies show that more than 80 of the cannabinoids that are found in the cannabis plant, both THC and non-THC, are responsible for relieving nausea and vomiting.

When CBD was used on rats in 2012, it was proven to decrease the nausea in rats. Furthermore, it was shown that, when used in humans, it decreases the need to vomit. However, if CBD is taken in an overdose, or just higher than normal doses, it can actually increase your risk of nausea—or have no effect on you at all.

Can Decrease Risk of Diabetes

According to a study from 2006, CBD can reduce the occurrence of diabetes in mice—taking the incidence of diabetes all the way down to 30 percent. This means that, if used correctly, with diet and exercise, it can actually heal the symptoms of diabetes and reverse it.

Furthermore, in a study back in 2013, the American Journal of Medicine stated that CBD and marijuana had an affect on glucose levels in the blood, along with insulin resistance. Studies showed that people who used marijuana and CBD had about 16% lower levels of insulin in their blood when they were fasting. This is a good sign, showing that your body can handle glucose better—and that you aren't spiking your insulin, which can lead to inflammation and ultimately other disorders related to diabetes, like heart disease.

Furthermore, this same study found a link between using marijuana and having a slimmer waist. As the fat around the mid section is specifically damaging, and ultimately leads to things like diabetes and even cancers, this is a huge find.

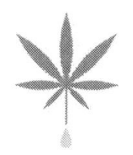

CHAPTER 4:
Buying CBD Oil: What You Need to Know

HOW TO GET CBD LEGALLY

At this current time, CBD is classified as a schedule one drug in the United States. This is because it's present in marijuana. This means, according to law, it has the potential to be abused and the potential to seriously affect your life.

However, medical research is changing that, as it looks into CBD and other marijuana ingredients. And in recent years, 17 states have voted in the utilization of lower-THC and higher-CBD medications and oils. Of course, each state has their own share of conditions in order for you to seek out CBD. This usually involves registering as a patient and ensuring that you're mentally healthy enough to handle CBD.

However, if you are legally allowed to get CBD products in your state, then look on for the top ways to take CBD oil—finding which one is best for you.

Different Varieties of CBD Oil

There are several different varieties of CBD oil. Even before deciding how you want to take it (we'll get into that later), there are several different strengths and packaging, all of which will affect how you treat yourself, medicinally or otherwise.

There are, essentially, three main types of CBD oil. All products generally fit into the following:

- *Raw CBD Oil*

- *Decarboxylated CBD Oil*

- *Filtered CBD Oil. This is commonly referred to as the "gold" line.*

The Raw CBD Oil is characterized by the following: it's in its original format, straight from the plant, without any processing beyond its first extraction. It will contain other raw ingredients, like lipids from the chlorophyll, bits of plant, and terpenes. The color of the Raw CBD oil will generally be a darker green, or even a black, and it will be thicker, as it isn't filtered down.

Generally, people who opt for Raw CBD oil want all the benefits of the cannabis plant, and not just the benefits from the CBD oil. It's generally purchased by people who are trying to use it to treat their insomnia, anxiety, or other mild issues like that.

Furthermore, Raw CBD oil is generally the cheapest, as it doesn't require the processing step. It has a lower amount of CBD, per volume, than the other two versions. Read on for that information below.

Decarboxylated CBD Oil is generally bought by those buyers who wish to make their own CBD edibles. They generally have mild problems, such as migraines and headaches, arthritis, anxiety, depression, or other ailments, and are looking to self-medicate.

Decarboxylated CBD oil is very similar to the Raw CBD oil, except that—as it states in the name—it's been decarboxylated. This process actually ups the "strength" of the CBD oil, making it work faster in the body. But what is this process, exactly? To put it simply, decarboxylation is a chemical reaction. It removes a carbon atom from the inside of the molecule, which turns CBDA into CBD—which fits better into the cell receptors in your brain and body.

Therefore, the "raw" version of CBD doesn't necessarily work alongside your body as readily (although it does offer the same benefits). Thusly, if you want more bang for your CBD buck, opt for decarboxylated. Much of the work has already been done for you.

Decarboxylated CBD oil is dark green or black, and, similar to the raw variety, is thick at normal temperature.

Unlike the "gold" filtered oils, decarboxylated oils are mid-grade price.

Filtered CBD Oil is the "gold variety," or highest-priced variety of CBD oil. It's actually the most frequently purchased across the United States, with people opting for it to treat everything from their anxiety, to their depression, to even worse ailments. This is generally the highest concentrated of all the possible CBD oils, as it's decarboxylated and then also filtered. This makes sure that the dark green plant chlorophyll is completely gone, along with lipids and other plant parts.

How Much CBD Oil Should You Take Per Day?

Several researchers and CBD oil specialists recommend taking a daily dose of around a tenth of a gram two times per day. However, this amount is always personal, depending on your individual preferences and how your body handles CBD oil.

When receiving the CBD oil as a concentrate (we'll talk more about the various ways to take CBD oil below), it's important to know that you could find yourself faced with a few different kinds of packaging. These includes syringes, plastic jars, or silicone jars. There are benefits to each of them, as well as drawbacks.

For one, a syringe is easiest for storing and dispensing CBD oil. However, when the syringe grows cold, the oil might have difficulty getting out of the syringe. However, you can easily warm up a syringe by placing it in warm water, or even placing it in a towel and heating it up in the microwave (for only a few seconds).

A plastic jar packaging will normally suit the "raw" CBD oil best. These are difficult for exact dosing, but can be used if you want to rub it on your skin or imbibe it with more convenience than the syringe.

The silicone jar is a brand new way of dispensing CBD oil, and it's most often used by people who want to "dab," or keep taking it throughout the entire day. The jars are easy to open and close, but unfortunately, many have found that they open up in the middle of walking, wasting the oil.

How Much CBD Is In Your Packaging?

In each gram, there is 1000 milligrams. Therefore, depending on the percentage of the CBD oil, you can calculate how many milligrams are found in each gram. If, say, you're dealing with 22.4% concentration of CBD in 1 gram, then that means you have 224 mg of CBD oil in that gram. If you're handling a syringe, it's incredibly easy to calculate, whereas, with other packaging, it can be more difficult.

Top Ways To Get Your CBD Oil

The benefits of CBD oil are absolutely incredible, backed by scientists all over the world. But there are countless options when purchasing your first CBC oil, which can make it confusing.

At this time, there are five general ways to take CBD oil. They're: as a topical, on your skin; as a tincture; as a capsule; as a vape; as a spray; or as a concentrate. Now, when purchasing these various things, it's essential to do your research. As with anything else, making a decision on a brand or product varies from product to product. We'll give you hints as much as we can going through it. But a poor product will normally have poor reviews—just like a bad blender from the internet, or a poor restaurant review.

CBD AS A CONCENTRATE:

Compared to other versions of CBD, CBD as a concentrate is of course more concentrated, and has the highest dose. It has more than ten times the concentration of the other products listed here. Plus, they're incredibly convenient, allowing you to consume them in just a couple seconds. And beyond that, they're not messy—which is always a plus.

Unfortunately, CBD as a concentrate isn't as "fun" as the others—if you care about that. They don't come in any flavors, which means the "natural" flavor is all you'll taste. Some people don't like that. Plus, concentrates look a bit scary if you're not used to them, as they look like needles.

To use the concentrates, simply eject the concentrate beneath your tongue and along the inside of your cheeks. Don't swallow it all at once. Simply allow it to be ingested into you very steadily. And then, allow the CBD to work its magic.

Note that the CBD as a concentrate is best utilized for those of us who are super busy, but who want the highest potency possible when imbibing.

CBD AS A TINCTURE

This is actually the most frequently used of all the versions of CBD oil. Like concentrate, tinctures don't separate the CBD oil, which makes it more pure. However, unlike CBD concentrate oil, tinctures can have a bit of flavor to them, which makes them more enjoyable.

These are taken much like concentrate. You simply drop a few drops beneath your tongue. This could get a bit messy, as the dropper isn't the most effectual, and the more regular user normally opts for concentrate, as it takes the "drippage" out of the equation.

CBD AS A CAPSULE

Of all the ways to take CBD oil, taking it as a capsule is the easiest. Which makes sense, of course. Pop it into your mouth, swallow it, and forget about it. It goes along with any vitamins you might currently take, or even any pills.

Each capsule of CBD offers around 10 to 25 mg of CBD. This allows you to keep track of your serving size, rather than having to calculate it in the tinctures or concentrates. However, if you're looking to gradually increase your CBD oil intake, then this makes the capsules a bit limiting. You always have to double your amount, or triple it. There's nothing gradual about it.

People normally resolve this issue by taking the capsules alongside other versions, like tinctures or concentrates, and gradually increase that way.

CBD OIL AS A SPRAY

Perhaps unsurprisingly, taking CBD oil as a spray is the weakest possible way to take it. The concentration is the lowest, as it must be more of a liquid to have the ability to spray. Typically, the concentration of a CBD spray is between 1 mg and 3 mg—which is absolutely nothing in comparison to the other varieties. Plus, because you're taking it orally, it's far more difficult to measure how much you're taking in. The sprays aren't always even, and you're left wondering.

However, that isn't to say CBD oil sprays aren't convenient and well-liked over a broad population of people. In fact, the sprays are very easy to carry in your pocket or in a purse. And it's much easier to just spray the oil in your mouth every once in a while, rather than hit up the tinctures or concentrates.

Typically, to spray it, spray about two or three times daily, or as much as you need to.

CBD OIL AS A TOPICAL

More and more CBD oil companies have begun offering CBD topical creams and salves and even lip balms, saying that they offer skin benefits. And in fact, CBD oils are actually shown to aid with things like psoriasis, acne, inflammation, anti-wrinkles, amongst others.

When you're opting for topical creams that purport they contain CBD oil, you should always ensure that the product uses encapsulation, or nano technology, or something called the "micellization" of the oil. This ensures that the CBD won't just remain on the top of your skin. Rather, it will dive below and actually interact with the cells you need it to.

When using topical CBD creams, it's essential to use it only when you feel it's necessary—when you really have a problem that requires this kind of solution. You can use it like lotion when you have dry skin, or when you have psoriasis. But don't apply it needlessly, all throughout the day. It'll be too much, and it'll be an overkill of the benefits.

CBD OIL TAKEN AS A VAPE

Compared to other methods, vaporizing the CBD through vape oil doesn't seem to lend as many benefits as tinctures or concentrates or even capsules. However, some other users of the CBD oil as vape oil say that smoking it is actually the most effectual way to get a more "even" absorption. This is because when you ingest things, it can lead to a delayed effect, depending on what else you've eaten that day.

Plus, when you smoke CBD vape oil, you can adjust the amount you take in based on how you feel immediately after.

In order to smoke the CBD oil, you'll need to invest in an e-cigarette or a vaporizer, or even just a vape pen. When you turn on the device, simply smoke it the way you might smoke a cigarette, and blow out the smoke.

BEYOND THE FIVE MAIN TYPES...

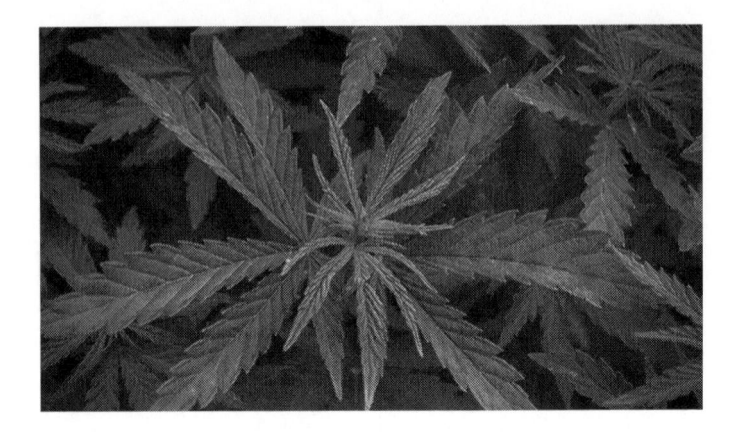

Beyond the types listed above, there are a few other ways to take CBD oil. These include: edibles, CBD patches, or even CBD gums. Among these, people are really picking up on the edibles. Unfortunately, unlike many of the other options—the tinctures, the concentrates—it's incredibly difficult to know just how much of the CBD oil you're ingesting with this edible. Sure, it might be delicious. But that isn't the real reason you're trying to eat it.

BEST BRANDS SELLING CBD OIL RIGHT NOW: A BREAKDOWN

These are the early days of CBD oils. The best possible brands to buy right now—reviewed by us based on their quality and prices as well as customer service—can help you make the best decisions.

DELTA BOTANICALS

This American brand utilizes only hemp that's grown in the States, making it locally-sourced. They offer several unique flavors. Plus, the tinctures can be used doubly as vape juice or as the droplets.

CW HEMP

CW Hemp is involved with a larger brand known as Charlotte's Web. This web is ultimately working alongside a young girl named Charlotte, who suffers from Dravet syndrome. They sell tinctures only, and their hemp is all grown in the United States.

MARY'S NUTRITIONALS

Mary's Nutritionals has several different varieties of topical creams and patches, along with sprays and tinctures. All of their stuff tastes like cinnamon, which is pretty fun. Unfortunately, they don't offer a very good online shopping experience.

HEMP MEDS

This brand offers everything from capsules to tinctures, to topical and concentrates. There's no genetic modification whatsoever, and they have zero chemical fertilizers or pesticides. Plus, they allow returns for online orders.

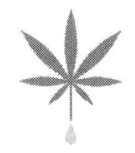

CHAPTER 5:
Extracting CBD and Making Your Own Hemp Oil

Did you know you can make your own hemp oil? As it's a beneficial part of any nutritional diet, having it around the house, homemade and ready for you, is never a bad thing. The essential fatty acids found in the hemp oil have been proven to have anti-inflammatory effects, due to their omega 3 fatty acids and their omega 5 fatty acids. Plus, it's just delicious when added to things like salad dressings, hummus, and pesto. But we'll handle that in a later chapter.

The preparation time for making hemp oil from the seeds is only 15 minutes, with the extraction time from the actual seeds depending on what kind of press you're using. With the recipe we're dealing with here, you will create approximately 80 grams of hemp oil from seeds.

The main ingredient you need is 4 cups of shelled hemp seeds.

It's essential to shell the hemp seeds, as the hull will just make extra work for the processor.

For the process, you'll also need: a home oil press, fuel for the lamp, a bottle lamp with a wick, a jar for taking in the oil, a lighter, and a bowl to take in the "trash" from the process.

Manual home oil presses kind of look like pasta makers, and operate in a similar way. The bottle lamp is down beneath the press, and the seeds are in a hopper on the top. You turn the crank to pass the seeds through the press, separating the oil.

FOLLOW ALONG WITH THESE STEPS:

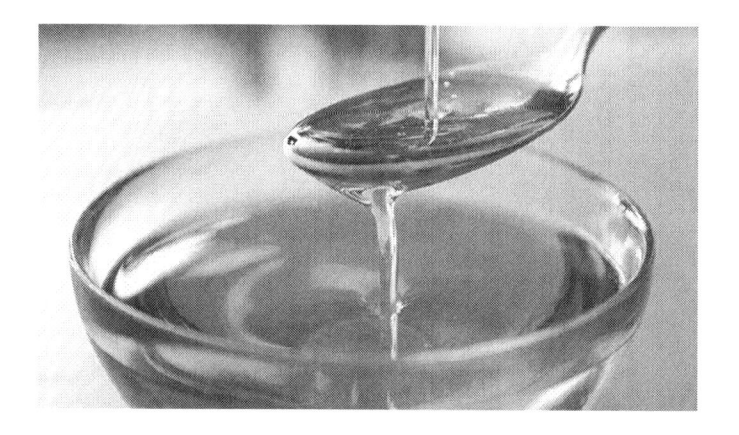

First, prep the press. Do this by securing the press to your countertop, unless you have someone to actually hold the press while you're pressing the seeds.

Set the lamp up beneath the press, and then light it with the lighter or matches.

Allow the press to heat for about fifteen minutes at this time.

Next, fill the hopper of the press about one third of the way up. Then, start to turn the hand crank slowly, without rushing it. As you crank it, the oil droplets should begin to fall into the jar you've set up for taking in the oil.

As the seeds grind, add more and more, but make sure not to overload the hopper. This would make it potentially clog.

When the hemp seeds have separated from their oil, they'll come out the other side really dehydrated and without use. You can use these seeds as compost in the garden, or you can just throw them out.

Repeat the process until you've completely run out of seeds.

Know that it's essential to clean up your press after pressing the oil, as you'll want to use it again. This piece of machinery is gentle, and if you want to use it again—you should take care of it.

HOW TO MAKE CBD OIL

Making CBD oil is another matter completely, generally speaking, CBD oil is bought from places that are government approved. Thusly, if you make your own, you're making a legal risk, as well as a physical one. If you do make it at home, it's recommended you only do it if you have your own medical marijuana license.

To make your own, you'll need the following:

2 plastic buckets

an ounce of marijuana, using a strain that has a higher amount of CBD (rather than focused on THC)

1 coffee filter

1 wooden stick

500 ml of isopropyl alcohol

a rice cooker

another large container

a fan, for ventilation

1 tsp. of water

a bowl or container that's stainless steel

a glass bottle

a dehydrator

With this recipe, you should be able to create about four grams of CBD oil, depending on the amount of CBD or THC that's in your strain.

Directions:

1. First, ensure that the marijuana and all other materials are completely dried. Place the marijuana in one of the plastic buckets.

2. Next, dampen the marijuana with the isopropyl alcohol. Next, crush the hemp using a wooden stick. The marijuana should crush in an even way, despite being slightly damp.

3. At this time, add more of the isopropyl alcohol until the marijuana is just covered. Then, stir it around using the wooden stick for about four minutes. At this point, the THC and CBD will be dissolving off of the marijuana and into the alcohol.

4. Pour the oil and the alcohol mixture into the second plastic bucket. Now add more alcohol to cover the marijuana, and then stir for an additional three minutes, using the wooden stick.

5. Next, add this mixture back into the other bucket. Toss out the plant, leaving only the oil and alcohol.

6. At this time, pour the mixture through the coffee filter, adding what remains to a clear container.

7. Next, you'll need your rice cooker in order to boil the solvent off. This is the slightly physically dangerous part, as the fumes from this process can be toxic and should not be breathed in. Therefore, set up the rice cooker in a space that's very well ventilated, and add a fan for good measure to blow out the fumes. Ensure that you don't put the rice cooker near anything like sparks or cigarettes or hot stoves, as that could make the fumes more powerful.

8. Fill the rice cooker to about three quarters of the way full. Plug the rice cooker in, and set it on the highest setting. The temperature shouldn't be any higher than 290 degrees Fahrenheit, or 140 degrees Celsius.

9. As the mixture drops more and more in the rice cooker, continue to add the remainder of the

alcohol solvent until the entire amount is in the rice cooker.

10. When the rice cooker holds only one inch of the mixture at the bottom, you'll need to add the one tsp. of water to the mixture. This will ensure that the oil doesn't completely overheat.

11. At this time, place oven mitts on your hands for safety reasons, and lift your rice cooker. Swirl it until the rest of the solvent evaporates into the air.

12. Next, pour the created solvent into the stainless steel bowl or container.

13. Add the stainless steel container into the dehydrator for three hours. This allows the rest of the solvent and the water to completely exit the oil.

14. When the oil has stopped its bubbling, you can add it to a clean bottle for storage and use it as you wish.

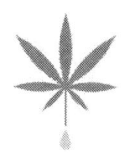

CHAPTER 6:

Beauty and Health Recipes With Hemp Oil

Hemp oil is one of the most nutritious ingredients to have in your kitchen, allowing for endless experimentation and gorgeous benefits. As mentioned, it contains an incredible amount of protein, along with omega-3 fatty acids and omega-6 fatty acids. This can help reduce cholesterol, help you lose weight, and fight against skin disorders like eczema and psoriasis, as well as simple things like pimples.

When using hemp oil in the kitchen, it's essential never to heat it, as this will change the unsaturated fats to saturated. Too much saturated fat can lead to heart disease, and other ailments, and thus negate all the benefits of hemp oil.

Instead, you can add hemp oil to recipes like: dips, salad dressings, hummus, smoothies, cold soups, and pesto. You should always opt for cold-processed, unrefined hemp oil, when purchasing, as this ensures it has retained its nutrients from the plant's seeds.

Check out the recipes below to add extra hemp to your diet.

HEMP OIL AND GARLIC DRESSING

Recipe Makes 8 Servings.

Preparation Time: 1 hour

Ingredients:

1/3 cup hemp oil

5 minced garlic cloves

1/3 cup white wine vinegar

1/4 tsp. pepper

1/4 tsp. salt

Directions:

Stir together the listed ingredients until well-mixed.

Allow the salad dressing to sit for one hour, ensuring that the garlic really gets into the liquid.

Then, shake the mixture well, and drizzle the dressing over your salad. Enjoy.

PESTO WITH HEMPSEED

Recipe Makes 6 Servings.
Preparation Time: 5 minutes

Ingredients:

5 tbsp. hemp oil

1/3 cup hempseed

2 1/4 cups Parmesan cheese, grated

5 minced garlic cloves

2 tsp. Sea salt

Directions:

First, add the ingredients to your food processor and blend until smooth. Taste the mixture, and season to your liking. Serve on salad or on bread, and enjoy.

CREAMY SALAD DRESSING WITH HEMP

Recipe Makes 1 cup.

Preparation Time: 10 minutes

Ingredients:

1/3 cup water

1/2 cup hemp seeds, hulled

2 tsp. hemp oil

2 tbsp. lemon juice

2 minced garlic cloves

1/2 tsp. Sea salt, or to taste

Directions:

Blend together the ingredients in a blender until smooth, adjusting the salt to taste. Then, add the dressing to a container, and allow it to chill in the fridge for about 20 minutes. This will allow the mixture to thicken.

HEMP SEED VINAIGRETTE FOR SALADS

Recipe Makes 3 Servings.

Preparation Time: 5 minutes

Ingredients:

3 minced garlic cloves

1 tsp. lemon juice

3 tbsp. hemp oil

2 tbsp. Dijon mustard

1 tbsp. Balsamic vinegar

1/2 tsp. salt

1/2 tsp. pepper

Directions:

Whisk together the listed ingredients until well mixed.

Then, adjust the salt and pepper to taste. Serve over the salad of your choice, and enjoy.

HEMP OIL HUMMUS

Recipe Makes 2 Servings.
Preparation Time: 5 minutes

Ingredients:
1 cup garbanzo beans
2 tbsp. hemp oil
2 minced garlic cloves
2 tsp. Tahini
1/2 tsp. salt
1/2 tsp. pepper

Directions:
Add all the ingredients to a food processor and process until completely smooth (or until you reach your desired consistency).

Serve over pita bread, with vegetables, or by itself.

HEMP AND CHOCOLATE SMOOTHIE

Recipe Makes 2 Servings.

Preparation Time: 5 minutes

Ingredients:

3 dates

2 cups almond milk

3 tbsp. hemp seeds

1 tbsp. hemp oil

3 tbsp. Cocoa powder

1 banana, frozen

1/2 tsp. Cinnamon

4 ice cubes

Directions:

Add the ingredients to a blender and blend until smooth. Serve in two chilled glasses, and enjoy.

PURPLE BERRY HEMP OIL SMOOTHIE

Recipe Makes 2 Servings.

Preparation Time: 5 minutes

Ingredients:

2 bananas

2 cups hemp milk

2 tsp. hemp oil

1 tsp. Wheatgrass powder

1 tsp. chia seeds

1/2 tbsp. honey

1 tsp. vanilla

1 tsp. Flaxseed meal

1/2 tsp. sea salt

2 cups mixed berries, frozen

Directions:

Toss the ingredients into your blender and blend until smooth or until your desired consistency.

GREEN HEMP OIL SMOOTHIE

Recipe Makes 1 Servings.

Preparation Time: 5 minutes

Ingredients:

1 cup coconut water

1 banana, frozen

1 1/2 cups mango, frozen

1/3 cup Greek yogurt, plain

1 1/2 cups kale leaves

1 tbsp. hemp seeds

2 tsp. hemp oil

2 dates, without the pits

Directions:

Add the listed ingredients to a blender and blend until you reach your desired consistency. Enjoy.

HEMP OIL FOR BEAUTY AND SKIN CARE

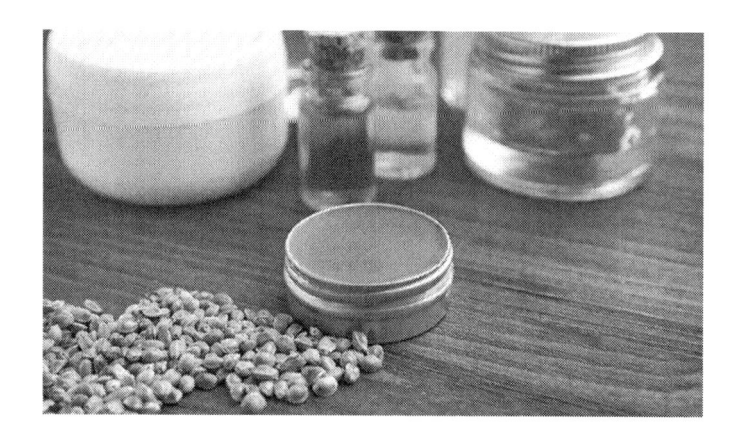

As mentioned in previous chapters, hemp oil, cultivated from the seeds of the hemp plant, is incredibly healthy for your skin, and is therefore utilized in many different skincare and beauty regimes.

Hemp oil allows for firmer and tighter skin, while adding extra antioxidants to fight things like inflammation, which can then lead to an increased appearance of wrinkles. It can further allow for longer-lasting moisturizing, which ensures that your skin retains its youthful glow throughout the day.

Furthermore, hemp oil can both calm irritated skin, as well as balance out any oily skin—making sure that it doesn't clog your pores or lead to pimples or acne.

Hemp oil is also able to take on most skin types, even the more sensitive ones, and can even be used for hair care, and it's incredibly "conditioning" in nature.

ESSENTIAL WAYS TO USE HEMP OIL FOR YOUR BEAUTY REGIME

Unlike much of your beauty supplies, hemp oil is relatively inexpensive (and pretty easy to make, if you use our recipe in a previous chapter). You can use it for countless things—one essential product—instead of buying a ton of different things to fill your medicine cabinet.

You can even use it to remove makeup.

There's a rule in the beauty world called "like dissolves like." And in this case, this works incredibly well. The hemp oil is similar to a lot of your makeup, like the oils and waxes in your eye makeup. In order to remove it, simply dab a bit of the oil with a cotton ball and remove the makeup slowly and tenderly.

You can use hemp oil to reduce your dry skin and heal it.

In order to do this, you just simply rub the hemp oil directly on the cracks in your skin. You can even do this for your feet and hands—massaging the oil into the cracked bits of skin and then donning either socks or gloves as you sleep. This will allow your skin to heal overnight, taking on the moisture of the oil.

Boost the health of your nails and cuticles.

If you have trouble with hangnails or just weak nails, you can rub the oil around your cuticles daily to boost their growth and strengthen them.

Make a skin facial.

In order to do this, cleanse your face, dry it, and then massage one tablespoon of the hemp oil all over your face. Then, place a warm, wet washcloth over the top of your face, allowing it to sit on your face until it cools. Then, wipe down your face with a washcloth, and repeat the process with an additional hot washcloth until all of the hemp oil is washed off. You don't need to wash your face after this, as it could just dry it out.

Use it to condition your hair.

Just before you use your shampoo in the shower, simply add about a tablespoon of hemp oil all over your scalp and allow it to sit on your head for about eight minutes. Afterwards, add the shampoo to your hair and wash like normal. Many women who do this actually don't need to condition their hair any longer!

Use it to fight your acne problems.

In order to do this, simply massage the hemp oil into your "problem" areas in your face, doing so for several minutes. While you do this, the hemp oil removes the "sebum plugs" within your skin, the stuff that causes cysts, blackheads, and whiteheads. You can do this every single day or during bad breakouts.

Rub it into eczema or psoriasis.

Jut as it does with acne and pimples, hemp oil has an ability to reduce symptoms of more serious skin disorders, like eczema. Simply rub about a tablespoon over the damaged area, every single day, and wait. This is much less chemical than your traditional over the counter medications, and therefore doesn't add anything "extra" toxic to the body.

Read on for some hemp oil-based recipes to use for self-care.

ANTI-ECZEMA HEALING BODY BUTTER

Ingredients:

1 ounce Shea butter

3/4 ounce hemp oil

3/4 ounce oat oil

3/4 ounce beeswax

Directions:

Melt the ingredients over low heat, being careful not to overheat as hemp oil can scorch very quickly and very easily.

After it's melted, pour the mixture into a clean container and allow it to harden into a body butter-consistency before applying to your skin.

FOREST FOR THE TREES BALM

Ingredients:

1/5 ounce beeswax

1/5 ounce bayberry wax

1 ounce safflower oil

1/4 ounce hemp oil

14 drops fir essential oil

6 drops spruce hemlock essential oil

10 drops white spruce essential oil

2 drops rose absolute

5 drops pine essential oil

Directions:

First, melt together the bayberry wax, hemp seed oil, beeswax, and the safflower oil in a small-sized double boiler. You can create your own double boiler by boiling a pot of water, and placing a smaller pot over the top of the water.

After the oils have melted together, remove the mixture from the heat. Add the essential oils, and stir slowly. Then pour the mixture into a tin, and allow it to set before using.

HEALING LIP BALM

Ingredients:

1/3 ounce beeswax

1/3 ounce jojoba oil

1/4 ounce Shea butter

1/5 ounce tamanu oil

1 tsp. vitamin E oil

1/5 ounce hemp oil

1 tsp. sunflower lecithin

1/3 ounce safflower oil

20 drops lavender essential oil

Directions:

First, add the beeswax, jojoba oil, and the safflower oil to a small double boiler and allow it to melt together. Stir well, and remove the mixture from the heat.

Next, add the rest of the ingredients: Shea butter, tamanu oil, vitamin E oil, hemp oil, and the sunflower lecithin, and stir well.

Afterwards, add the lavender essential oil, and pour the mixture into lip balm tubes. Allow it to set before using.

HEMP OIL FACE MASK WITH AVOCADO

Ingredients:

1 avocado

2 tbsp. Bentonite clay

4 tbsp. hemp oil

5 drops lemongrass essential oil

1 1/2 tbsp. coconut oil

Directions:

First, add the avocado—peeled and cored, of course, hemp oil, coconut oil, and the essential oil to a blender or a food processor, and process the mixture until smooth.

Then, pour the mixture into a bowl, and add the clay, using your hands to really mix it up.

Next, apply the mixture to your face. Leave the mask on your face for fifteen minutes before rinsing it off and patting your face dry.

HEMP OIL SOAP

Ingredients:

5 ounces coconut oil

5 ounces olive oil

5 ounces hemp oil

2 ounces lye

3/4 ounces lavender essential oil (or whatever essential oil you like best)

6 ounces water, distilled works best

Directions:

First, realize that making soap is a bit different than the other "get it hot and stir" scenarios. Make sure you use goggles, gloves, and wear shirts with longer sleeves.

Heat the water to boiling, and add the lye to the water. Stir this mixture, making sure not to breathe in. Next, set this mixture to the side and allow it to cool down to around 110 degrees Fahrenheit.

Next, stir together the oils. Allow them to melt in a double boiler, and then allow them to cool to around 110 degrees Fahrenheit as well (within five degrees of the water and lye).

Next, add the lye and water to the oils, slowly. Then, stir the mixture very quickly, until it looks like a thin pudding. This could take a while if you don't use something like an immersion blender.

Next, pour the soap into your molds and allow them to sit at room temperature for five days. Then, remove them from the molds, and allow them to cure for six weeks before using.

Printed in Great Britain
by Amazon